The Fit Man

The ABC's of Fitness
For
Mind and Body

I0435477

RON KNESS

Contents

Fitness: The Missing Piece of the Puzzle?

Congrats on starting a workout plan! For the first time, or fifth. If you're completely new to working out, you will soon become amazed by the changes your body is capable of and hopefully become an avid iron enthusiast.

The truth is, we all desire a good body. Moreover, it comes with many perks, far beyond what you see when you look at a chiseled six-pack and bulging arms. If done safely, you've just added years to your life!

Training shouldn't be rocket science - when it boils down to it, your body knows what it needs. Do not become a victim of "analysis paralysis" trying every new routine that comes out!

Stick to the basics of performing full body, or exercises that utilize more than one muscle group and you will develop true functional fitness (those movements that translate well to the things you do every day in real life).

So, primed with your enthusiasm and a thirst for knowledge, let's dive straight into it!

Why Is General Fitness Important?

If you've never fallen seriously ill in your life, and find yourself questioning the necessity of good fitness, chances are that you've taken it for granted. In fact, the majority of adult men adapt a "wait and see" kind of approach in the sense that unless something seems wrong, it's just an additional chore.

Boy, do we men have a hell-bent mentality! It's true- women are more likely than men to have a fulltime gym membership, which they ACTUALLY USE, as opposed to the sterner sex. So, besides the obvious statement of improving overall health, what can improving your fitness do for you?

LOOK GREAT

Let's be realistic here fellas- chances are that most men start hitting the gym in an effort to become aesthetically pleasing to women. Luckily, most men realize after a few months (hopefully you get that far) that working out becomes a way of life, done for oneself, as opposed to for attention.

The change in body composition is unquestionable as you reduce body fat, build lean muscle mass, look denser and more ripped, and your clothes flatter your muscular shape, in short, you are a lean, mean, sexy machine.

Muscle is more compact than fat, even though it is heavier, so you get away with weighing more but give an illusion of being light.

IMPROVE DAILY PERFORMANCE

Sure, you may feel fine today, or even 10 years from now for that matter; but when the day of pain arrives, will you wish that you had taken advice and began working out? You bet your bottom you will!

The human body is a well-crafted machine that requires frequent work and maintenance. This applies particularly to the muscles and joints, which become atrophied from years of misuse (lack of). Frequent exercise makes this tissue more capable of load bearing, as is required in our day-to-day use of them.

Studies have demonstrated that regular physical activity started at a young age significantly reduces the chance of injury in later years, as well as joint and bone impairment (arthritis, osteoporosis). There is no better time than today to start an exercise and fitness program.

PUMP UP BRAIN POWER

Find yourself getting a little lax in the memory department? Not surprisingly, since as we age our brain capacity decreases, by natural death of brain cells. However, what if you found out that exercise and good fitness could help alleviate or even reverse the effects of cognitive decline? Of course, you'd be interested!

The Two Mechanisms Behind This Brain Boost Are:

- **Improving Blood Flow To The Brain:** reduced blood flow can lead to starvation/ poor perfusion of the cells in the brain, causing "hypoxia" known as oxygen starvation to occur, or essential nutrients not being made readily available for various processes. Exercise improves blood flow throughout the entire body, as demonstrated by thermal scans of the brain before and after exercise. The result? Improved brain activity and neuronal connections.

- **Creation Of New Cells:** this is an eye opener for many reasons, primarily because previously all researchers were able to tell us was that age related mental decline was normal and irreversible. While that is still true, new research has shown that you can stimulate the growth of new brain cells, and forge powerful interconnection with intense exercise sessions, in particular cardiovascular exercise. Therefore, with that knowledge in mind, it is entirely possible to retain your mental capacities well into old age.

PREVENT DISEASE

Would you be surprised that the majority of diseases and illnesses that occur in the developed world are non-communicable? That refers to diseases that cannot be caught from another individual, but primarily from lifestyle choices, and to a lesser degree, genetic. This is the so-called "rich man's" curse, whereby situations of excess are responsible for health decline, as opposed to infections from pathogens.

The Best Way To Combat Non-Communicable Diseases?

A well thought out fitness plan with a sensible diet. Exercise alone will yield significant results, but if the avoidance of disease is your goal, diet must become an integral part of your lifestyle.

You Can Significantly Reduce Your Chance Of Developing:

- Heart disease, including stroke, and heart failure
- High blood pressure
- Type 2 diabetes
- Obesity
- Depression
- Various types of cancer
- Osteoporosis

And many more conditions! The evidence is overwhelming; general fitness is a mandatory pre-requisite to a long, disease free and productive life.

The Importance of Muscle

Chances are you do not have any interest in becoming as massively muscular as professional bodybuilders become and that's understandable.

Why? Primarily because the body does not naturally achieve those levels of muscularity. It requires administration and ingestion of tons of drugs, ranging from steroids, growth hormone, to insulin and many other hardcore drugs that are indicated for medical conditions. Honestly, unless you plan to aim for the professional leagues, the risk of damage to your body is far too great. Many casual gym-goers are now on some form of drug, with not much to be expected except a good body.

However, this is not to de-emphasize the importance of carrying decent muscle on your frame. Muscle is quite likely among the top four structural components in the body, being responsible for ensuring your body is kept upright and easily facilitates various motions.

Moreover, as you may have noticed with an older relative or friend, "use it or lose it." Muscles are likely to atrophy if not used in a manner conducive to their growth, strengthening, or maintenance. By this, we mean resistance based exercise.

Sure, walking is universally good, but it is unlikely to do much for your muscles in terms of strength or functionality. Have you ever stopped to compare an endurance runner with a sprint athlete? Why is it that one has scrawny, tiny muscles, while the other has massive muscular development, often without use of drugs? It is because of the stress requirements placed on that body.

Type 1 Versus Type 2 Muscle Fibers

Low intensity endurance athletes have highly developed type 1 muscles fibers; which come into play during periods of low intensity, endurance based exercises. Think of a slow job for many miles. Whereas, athletes whose disciplines require a high degree of power/ speed output, have well developed type 2 muscle fibers.

The difference?

Type 2 muscle fibers are much larger (think of engine size) and are capable of eliciting rapid changes to speed or power (think of sprinting), whereas type 1 fibers are recruited for low intensity day to day movements (typing, walking, lifting a spoon to your mouth).

Type 2 muscle fibers carry the best potential for strength development, and this is why they are much more important in maintaining the structural integrity of your body for years to come.

Muscle mass is responsible for a range of functions detailed below.

MAINTAINING YOUR POSTURE

One of the most under-appreciated roles of muscle is in the maintenance of good posture. The muscles of the back and abdominal regions, especially, contribute significantly to spinal health and avert your osteoporosis risk as you age. If you have a job that requires hours of sitting at a desk, you will appreciate the benefits of a healthy posture, as you will not experience back pain and other joint related issues of the spine.

OBESITY PREVENTION

Did you know that people who carry higher amounts of muscle mass are less likely to become obese? This is simply because of the metabolic requirements of muscle as they help you to expend more calories even at rest.

In addition, you're likely to experience an even greater "afterburn" following an intense weight lifting session. Lean muscle mass simply helps you get lean faster.

INCREASED ENERGY LEVELS

Did you know that by design our metabolism is primarily fat based?

Yes, primitive man consumed a diet that was high in saturated animal fat and protein, and yet remained extremely lean.

Our modern day diet has FORCED a metabolic change to sugars, which even though important to the brain, were well off with fat being the primary energy source back then.

Fat is a more efficient energy source for two reasons:

- Its caloric density is double that of a gram of protein or carbohydrate, each gram of fat liberates 9 calories, while the other two supply just 4calories/gram. In addition, fat does not result in the roller coaster ride that is insulin release, or does so in a much more controlled fashion.

- Carbs are not efficiently stored, is it any surprise that our bodies can only store a small amount of carbs at a time? In comparison to fat, which our muscles readily accept as energy currency, and which is the preferred storage.

This muscle supporting diet results in naturally higher levels of lean body mass, since in addition to working out hard, diet must be on point.

BONE DENSITY CORRELATES TO MUSCLE MASS

You've probably heard this statement spewed around repeatedly, but have you ever taken the time to question why?

It has to do with actual load bearing potential. Larger muscles have a higher capacity for carrying weight, which translate to stronger bones as well. Think about it, the best way to strengthen bones is to increase the amount of load they can bear.

IMPROVE RECOVERY AFTER DISEASE

Muscle stores can act as a safety store for the body in times of serious illness or injury. Chances are that you will be on a subsistence diet at that time, consisting of the bare essentials to keep you alive. As such, your protein consumption drops way below required, which can hamper your recovery big time. Having large protein stores during such a phase allows speedy recovery of the body.

The importance of maximizing your lean muscle mass cannot be emphasized enough.

The Premise of Fat Burning

Chances are that you've tried a "fat loss" diet at some point in time, and were fed up when you did not achieve proper results. However, it was more than likely that you were not giving 100% to your end goal, or maybe even skipped exercise altogether!

Dieting is exceptionally important for long-term weight loss, but it is unlikely to make your body more efficient at fat loss, without constantly reducing calories and modifying caloric intakes, there is a better way.

Train To Improve Your Fat Burning Machinery: Muscle

In fact, knowledge of how to best optimize your body composition, leading to the most significant fat loss has changed significantly over the past 20 years.

In the past, fat burning was based on doing slow and boring cardio workouts to burn off a fairly low amount of calories in the moment, with none of the post workout fat burning potential that can be obtained through high intensity workouts that are both shorter and much more efficient. This is just one method that promotes fat burning nirvana, as there are others.

MAKE RESISTANCE TRAINING THE BASE OF YOUR FITNESS PROGRAM

Hands down, the most efficient way to blow fat out of the water (well, your body in this case) is to increase the amount of muscle cells (hyperplasia) as well as their size (hypertrophy) your body has on its frame.

Why?

Because muscle burn fat, as they require massive amounts of calories for maintenance and sustenance that quickly add up to become fat annihilators. In addition, the afterburn following weight training (known in nerdy circles as EPOC, or exercise post oxygen consumption) leads to tons of calories being used up in an effort to reinitiate muscle synthesis, and blunts fat gain for a period of time.

Still think those guys are muscle heads?

FOCUS ON HIGH-INTENSITY INTERVAL TRAINING

Which brings us to the second most important component of training, high intensity. As previously mentioned, gone are the days (or they should be gone) when slow low intensity cardio prevailed since today the science is clear and has revealed that performing intervals of very high effort, alternated with lower intensity recovery periods, are much more efficient at burning fat OVER THE LONG HAUL.

This is an important distinction to be made, since if you compare low intensity with high intensity cardio side by side, you will likely be fooled by the results. It would demonstrate better fat burning in the low intensity group, immediately following training. However, it stops there, because as soon as exercise is completed, fat burning stops!

This is not so for HIIT (high intensity interval training), since there is a similar after burn experience as seen in weight training.

The result?

You burn more calories over 24 hours doing absolutely nothing, as opposed to short-term higher burn in the low intensity group.

RON KJNESS

The morale of this story is stop doing an hour of monotonous cardio and start doing 15 minutes of HIIT!

DON'T DISCOUNT THE IMPORTANCE OF NUTRITION

It has been seen too often, guys who give 95% in the gym, and only 5% towards their diets. That is why they work so hard, and have little to show for it.

The simple reality is that your diet can easily be responsible for 70% of the progress you make, resulting in this factor actually being the most important.

When it comes to training for lean muscle gain, what you eat is just as important as WHEN you eat. For example, at most times throughout the day insulin is quite the nuisance, it preferentially shuttles your ingested calories to be stored as fat (the excess calories) and will not shuttle to muscle unless an anabolic stimulus is in place.

Upon waking, and before hard training sessions, meals that are rich in both carbohydrates and proteins are optimal, with fat being reduced to the minimum. However, at other times of the day, your preferred meals should be high protein/ moderate fat and veggies, to purposefully facilitate the burning of fat as fuel.

16

Muscles need to be fed, if there is not a readily available source of carbohydrate, it goes to fat's high capacity stores. Over time, the body becomes extremely efficient at using fat for energy, so the initial bouts of lethargy and cravings become a thing of the past.

LOW INTENSITY CARDIO

Low intensity cardio still has a place in fitness plans, primarily as a backup, however. Steady state cardio is useful in periods following acute overtraining, or as a recuperative aid following a loading phase.

Ideally, training should be planned in 12-week cycles, followed by a week or two of "deconditioning," which allows the nervous system and muscles to equilibrate back to their normal state. Slow cardio can be used during these periods when your goal is "just to get some exercise in."

The Dreaded Belly Fat

The classic beer belly, we all know someone or quite a few who has this characteristic telltale sign of unhealthy fat storage, or more correctly; how many people do you know who DON'T have belly fat?

Why have the past few decades seen such an upsurge in men with potbellies, even though overall they might be as skinny as a twig?

Well, for one thing, chances are that they do not partake in exercise of any type. It is not unusual for slim men to believe that they are fit, when in reality they may be a hormonal time bomb.

THE DANGERS OF BELLY FAT

Belly fat, also known as visceral fat is the most dangerous type of fat in the body because it surrounds vital organ. Excess fat around the middle increases risk of premature death even in those who are not overweight, as shown in research published on Nov. 10 in the Annals of Internal Medicine, the risk is specific to men with a waistline that measures 40 inches or more.

Belly fat is also linked to stroke, diabetes, high cholesterol, and inflammation.

ELEVATED LEVELS OF STRESS HORMONES

Stress hormones are needed to help get us through very basic situations, such as prepping in time for the 8AM commute, or waking up in the morning. However, with this secretion of stress hormone, primarily cortisol, your body is signaled to "store for hard times" in this case, hog calories floating around in case a famine rolls out in a day or two. It is the way we were prehistorically wired to survive. In times of scarcity, man had to adapt or die.

As it relates to muscle, there is a definite connection between muscle mass and cortisol levels, higher cortisol levels corresponding to lower muscle mass. The hormones testosterone and cortisol also share opposite sides of the same coin, whereas testosterone favors anabolism and growth of new tissue, cortisol is catabolic that is destroying all but the necessary for survival. Secondarily, more muscle mass is likely to favor use of fat as fuel, thus promoting breakdown of excess belly fat.

This is not to say that you should not reduce stress levels as much as possible to eliminate excess cortisol levels that have been shown in research to promote increases in belly fat.

YOUR DIET IS FULL OF JUNK

This should be the most obvious reason why you have those massive potbellies, but specifically you are likely not consuming enough quality protein, and chicken nuggets are not your best choice.

Protein, in addition to stimulating muscle growth, in itself results in a high degree of calorie burning to ensure efficient digestion. This translates to less calories in per day, making it less likely that you store too many calories in your abdominal region.

Secondly, carbs can spike insulin levels massively, resulting in fat cells happily upping their storage via the cortisol connection. Protein blunts the peak insulin spike, making it less likely (or measurable) that the same amount of fat gain occurs.

Finally, sugars have the ability to retain water, which can worsen a bloated abdomen, or even worse, wheat based products may lead to intestinal discomfort, fermentation and diarrhea!

The bottom line?

Sugar can worsen your belly fat conundrum too many ways to mention. Eliminate sweets, table sugar, fruit juices, soda, and too much fruit pronto!

YOU DON'T WORKOUT

Initially, exercise seems like a stressful scenario and, you are right. Typically, high stress means increased cortisol and subsequent body fat storage.

HOWEVER, what makes exercise beneficial in your quest for washboard abs is multi-faceted, and quite easily overtakes the one possible (and unlikely) scenario of increased cortisol release.

Here's How:

- **Exercise Causes Release Of Endorphins:** These natural hormones/ chemicals made by the body are nature's way of relaxing and combating stress. They have an inherent effect on reducing cortisol levels, hence why you've likely heard exercise is a good method of stress relief of use in the treatment of depression.

- **Exercise Stimulates Growth Hormone And Testosterone Release**: Testosterone and growth hormones are potent natural anti-catabolic hormones, which blunt the effect of cortisol on the body.

Performed a few times weekly, exercise will, in addition to helping you lose weight via building of muscle/ burning calories, help you manage stress better, and offset the much hated accumulation of belly fat.

Endurance/Stamina/Strength: Triple Threat Advantage

If you've been actively partaking in a fitness program for any reasonable amount of time, you may find yourself spinning wheels going from objective to objective. What objectives? Either training for strength, endurance, or stamina.

However, a good fitness program SHOULD incorporate aspects of all these models, but should be measurable in one direction at a time.

First things first, do you understand exactly what these training goals are? In case you don't, here's a quick explanation:

- **Strength:** strength refers to the maximum resistance a muscle can bear. Bodybuilding and Olympic weightlifting are considered strength movements, since they seek to improve the amount of weight a muscle car bear over time. If you find yourself trying to increase the amount of weight you can lift over time, you are primarily emphasizing strength development.

- **Stamina:** wouldn't you love to be able to perform at max output for a longer period of time? We all would, that's a given. The time you can perform at your max, is referred to as your stamina. Therefore, in theory if you can bench press 200lbs, for a period of 20 seconds, that is your stamina. However, another person who can only bench 100lbs, but safely for 30 seconds, possesses higher stamina than you do. This is because both of you are performing at your limit, but the second person can perform at their maximum for longer. Similarly, sprint athletes constantly work on improving stamina, since being able to run at peak speed for a longer time is highly desirable.

- **Endurance:** ever seen athletes who can work out for seemingly hours on end, even though the intensity is sub-par? That is your typical endurance athlete. The major difference between stamina and endurance, is endurance's primary goal of maximal time (regardless of the low intensity), whereas stamina seeks maximal output for the maximal possible duration.

Now with a basic understanding of what these parameters represent, is it possible to simultaneously develop all three?

It most definitely is!

By utilizing a combination of strength movements (such as squats, presses and rows) with endurance exercises, such as jogging or low intensity cycling and stamina building movements (jump squats, wind assisted resistance sprints) it is possible to become proficient in all aspects of fitness.

Exercise and Disease Prevention

There are many possible reasons you may have begun working out in the first place, whether it be for the aesthetics, improving lean mass accrual, or reducing body fat; one thing that frequently accompanies your routine is a significant improvement of your health, and with it your resistance to disease.

A sound fitness program helps to reduce the likelihood of you developing many debilitating, non-communicable diseases, ensuring you enjoy a long high quality life.

Need more convincing? If you have family history of any of the following, or simply want to lower your risks, get started on a program ASAP.

OSTEOPOROSIS

A crippling disease that works by making bones "softer" or more brittle, leading to weakened structural support and increased likelihood of fractures.

About 2 million men are currently diagnosed with osteoporosis as cited by the National Osteoporosis Foundation. As many as 1 in 4 men age 50 or older who have this disease will break a bone, and approximately 12 million more men are at risk.

According to the International Osteoporosis Foundation, approximately, 20 to 25% of hip fractures occur in men, with an overall mortality rate of about 20% in the first year following a hip fracture. Additionally, while women are afflicted with this disease at higher rates than men are, men's mortality rates following a fracture are higher. The mortality rates from fractures also increase with age.

The residual lifetime risk of experiencing an osteoporotic fracture in men over the age of 50 is about 27%, which is higher than the 11.3% risk of developing prostate cancer, a leading cancer in men.

In addition to having a definite dietary connection, osteoporosis can also be prevented, or slowed down significantly by incorporating resistance training into their fitness plan.

Performed 3 times a week, people who weight train have higher bone densities and fewer instances of pain related to the spine.

BLOOD PRESSURE

Exercise, in addition to being a potent stress reliever, can help reduce blood pressure via a different mechanism; blood vessel dilation.

Many hypertensives have chronically tightened blood vessels, which exacerbate the likelihood of a cardio-ischemic event occurring, such as a stroke. Relaxation of blood vessels improves blood flow, and reduces resistance of blood in the vessels.

TYPE 2 DIABETES

Type 2 diabetes is at epidemic levels, with 90% to 95% of all diabetes cases being type 2, a preventable form that is mainly tied to lifestyle choices, like diet and exercise.

Men have a slightly higher risk of developing type 2 diabetes than women, though weight, age, belly fat, lack of exercise and poor diet are the most significant risk factors for the illness.

Exercise and sound fitness habits help you maintain a healthy weight, which greatly reduces your risk factors for getting this life threatening disease.

Resistance training can also significantly improve your sensitivity to insulin, resulting in less being able to work more efficiently. In case you don't know, the lower insulin is in the blood, the better it is for fat metabolism, overall energy, and health.

In addition, the recovery of muscle cells is very calorically intensive making sugars in the blood be shuttled into the muscles. Your body becomes better at partitioning nutrients for important functions, as opposed to fat storage.

DEPRESSION

Just because signs of this debilitating disease may not be physically visible, it does not mean that it is any less of a menace on society. In depression, there is an imbalance of hormones in different parts of the brain, resulting in poor responses to pleasure, or happiness.

The euphoria or "feel good" that comes from working out is because of an increase in endorphins; the chemicals in the body that relieve stress, and improve wellbeing and mood. In addition, since many people suffering from depression do not have suitable outlets for stress or leisure, getting started with a fitness routine can be just what the doctor prescribed.

HEART DISEASE

Quite likely, the most measurable impact that exercise has in disease prevention is that associated with heart disease. In individuals with poor health, the tiny blood vessels of the heart become more and more blocked over time, with plaque like residue called atherosclerotic deposits. These deposits narrow the inside diameter of these blood vessels, making it harder and harder for your heart to receive blood and oxygen, causing stabbing heart pains as time progresses, and increasing the likelihood of a major heart attack.

Following a heart attack, a part of the heart muscular wall becomes irreparably damaged, compromising the functioning of the heart.

Even though atherosclerotic plaques cannot be removed "per se," a good fitness plan, inclusive of resistance and cardiovascular training, can strengthen the heart muscles, help to initiate development of new blood vessels supplying the heart, and slowly but surely, delay your previously inevitable outcome of a heart attack.

The more you elevate your heart rate and work your heart during fast-paced exercise the stronger it becomes, therefore serving you as you age.

Fitness As You Age: Training for the Senior Man

Good fitness habits should be integrated and developed at a young age to ensure good health throughout life and as a measure of prevention as you get older. However, it is never too late to start working out, so if you are behind the times, and up in age, you can still do your body good by getting to the gym immediately.

For older men, cardio, strength training, balance and functional fitness workouts are recommended. If you are ready to get started consider your level fitness when choosing exercises and get a doctor's clearance.

Should a young man and older man train the same? Theoretically, no, they should not.

Why?

Because it is a natural part of aging for body structures to begin breaking down, or simply a case of them not being able to support the same load as a younger man.

But - and it's a big but - if you had started a fitness plan in your youth, and are merely trying to continue into your golden years, chances are you will be much more capable of going toe to toe with a younger man, than of you started for the first time in your life at age 55.

With that in mind, of course, there are guidelines, which you should keep in mind to remain injury free and active for years to come.

BE CONSCIOUS OF YOUR RECOVERY ABILITY

It's old news, the older you are, the slower your recovery becomes. So, do not attempt to perform intense exercise 5 days a week. Instead, aim for a more balanced 2 days per week of resistance training; working the entire both on days with sufficient rest between them (such as on Monday and then Thursday). By doing this, you allow your body enough time to recover from the previous session's workout.

In addition, perform low to moderate intensity cardiovascular exercise, using low impact methods. Best options including swimming, elliptical training, or cycling.

SET REALISTIC AND ATTAINABLE GOALS

If you're over 50, you will not gain pounds of lean mass every month, nor will you lose weight extremely fast. In fact, your body probably favors fat storage, and your metabolism is likely in pre-retirement. So, don't be disappointed if you do not make progress as fast as you'd expect, especially if you're new to training.

Your testosterone levels are weaning, as is growth hormone. Insulin sensitivity is likely poorer, and you may have concomitant diseases. Try to focus on consistency first, then let intensity follow.

STRETCHES ARE NOW MANDATORY

No longer can you get away with lackluster or no stretches at all, at this point in time, stretches are necessary to keep you injury free, and to properly warm up joint, muscles and tendons and signal that more work is coming. Post exercise static stretching is also helpful for seeding up recovery and decreasing intensity of DOMS (delayed onset muscle soreness), which typically occurs a day or two after training.

EAT ENOUGH

Have you ever noticed that typically, as you age your appetite, or the amount you can consume at one sitting is reduced? This is not necessarily a bad thing, but can become a problem in seniors when muscle atrophy accelerates and a mediocre diet becomes insufficient (actually leading to dietary deficiencies).

In such a scenario, there are two options:

- **Supplement With An Appetite Stimulant** - these come in various types, be it prescription or over the counter, and work to improve appetite. Depending on your physical needs, you can take it either once or twice daily, to maximize your intake of calories through the day

- **Eat Calorie Heavy Foods** - consume solid meals, loaded with protein and moderate amounts of good fat, and with low to moderate forms of slow digesting, fibrous carbs. Doing so ensures that whatever is eaten is rich in nutritive value, and will be used for muscular synthesis and recovery. Consumption of a complete multi-vitamin/multi-mineral is also be advised to ensure micro nutritional deficiencies do not develop.

Conclusion

Fitness is the catalyst to the change initiated by a solid diet. You can compare following a diet plan without fitness to a car being supplied premium quality gas and lubricants, but not being serviced to improve/change its parts. The body is similar, as it needs to be maintained by partaking in regular exercise, which strengthens many structural components, and also promotes internal efficiency (AKA metabolism).

If you truly wish to live your life to the fullest, be sure to mold a lifestyle that incorporates solid fitness practices. You only have one life, make it count.

Other Senior Health and Fitness Books by This Author

If you would like to read more about Senior Health and Fitness, here is a list of the titles, CreateSpace links and descriptions:

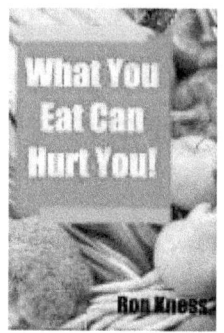

What You Eat Can Hurt You

https://www.createspace.com/4963196

Do you know that certain foods increase your risk for inflammation, disease and illness? It's true! And certain foods can help cure and heal you if you do get sick. Knowing which foods to eat and which ones to avoid empowers you to manage your own health.

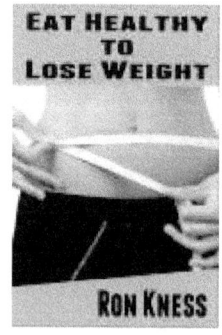

Eat Healthy to Lose Weight

https://www.createspace.com/4962939

As you read through our book, we show you which foods you should and should not be eating to reach your weight loss goal, along with discussing how to maintain your weight loss and stay within a few pounds of your goal weight. Banish the weight you keep gaining back each time by learning how to live a healthy lifestyle.

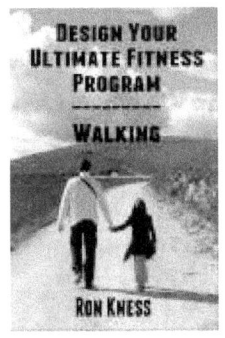

Design Your Ultimate Fitness Program - Walking

https://www.createspace.com/5252272

In my book Design Your Ultimate Fitness Program – Walking, we discuss the considerations that need to be made when designing a custom walking program, along with:

• Equipment needed
• Wearable technology you can use to track your walking
• And how to make walking more challenging

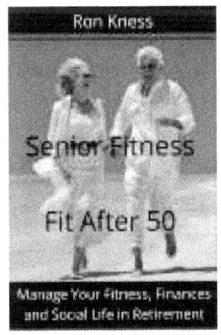

Senior Fitness – Fit After 50: Learn How to Manage Your Fitness, Finances and Social Life in Retirement

https://www.createspace.com/5474751

Inside you will discover answers to your most pressing questions:
• What do I need to know about downsizing my home?
• What are the best tips for staying healthy as you approach your 50's?
• When should I start planning for retirement?
• I am worried about being lonely once I retire, do others feel the same?

• Is it worthwhile to carry two homes during retirement? And more…

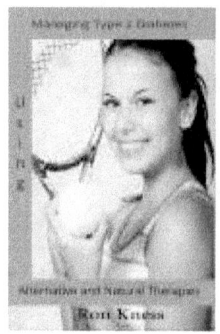

Managing Type 2 Diabetes Using Alternative And Natural Therapies

https://www.createspace.com/5401244

While Type 2 diabetes can be managed medically, there are many alternative natural and holistic methods of therapy and treatment that can further enhance quality of life and minimize the effects of this disease. In this book, I discuss 12 different types, including yoga, reflexology and acupuncture to name just three.

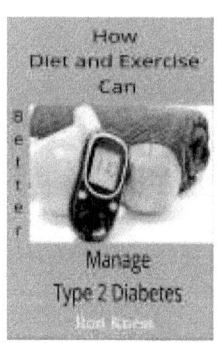

How Diet and Exercise Can Better Manage Type 2 Diabetes

https://www.createspace.com/5404845

Of the different types of diabetes, only Type 2 can be reversed. In my book How Diet and Exercise Can Better Manage Type 2 Diabetes, we reveal the three things you can do to best manage your disease, including:
• Diet
• Exercise
• Weight management

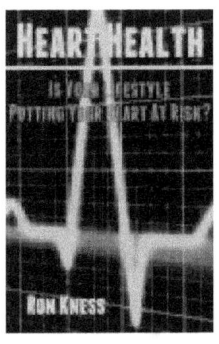

Heart Health: Is Your Lifestyle Putting Your Heart at Risk?

https://www.createspace.com/5464020

In my ebook Is Your Lifestyle Putting Your Heart At Risk? we discuss the six greatest risks to your heart and the lifestyle changes you can make to mitigate them.

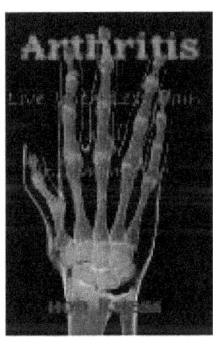

Arthritis – Live Wth Less Pain and Inflammation: Tips and Techniques You Can Use to Lessen the Pain and Inflammation

https://www.createspace.com/5457441

Discover Simple Tips & Information That Will Help Reduce The Painful Symptoms Of Arthritis!

You learn things like:
• Simple and effective information that will help you manage the pain and inflammation that comes along with arthritis, so that you can live an active, full life without debilitating pain.
• The different types of arthritis, their symptoms and how to alleviate their painful side effects.
• The pros and cons of over-the-counter arthritis medications, plus simple tips that will help you know how to choose the right supplements.

• Free, yet effective ways to get relief from arthritis pain and inflammation, so you don't have to suffer anymore.
the effects arthritis can have significant impact on your physical and mental well-being, but this books shows you how to overcome its painful symptoms and live life relatively pain free.

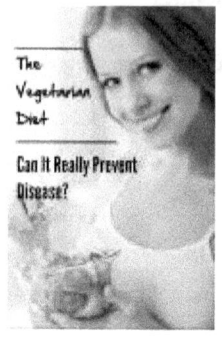

The Vegetarian Diet – Can It Really Prevent Disease?

https://www.createspace.com/5519874

Is a vegetarian diet right for you? Multiple studies have shown over and over that a vegetarian diet goes along way in preventing certain chronic diseases, such as:

• Heart Disease
• Cancer
• Diverticulitis
• Type 2 Diabetes
• Hypertension
• Obesity
• Kidney Failure

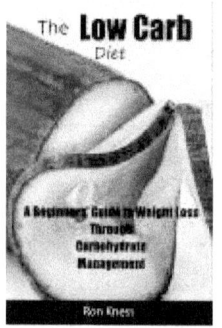

The Low Carb Diet: A Beginner's Guide to Weight Loss Through Carbohydrate Management

https://www.createspace.com/5416348

In my book "The Low-Carb Diet – A Beginners' Guide to Weight Loss Through Carbohydrate

Management", I reveal a successful method of losing weight based in part on the amount and type of carbohydrates you consume.

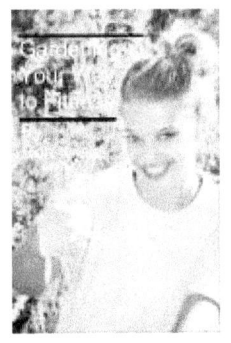

Gardening Your Way to Fitness: The Fun Way to Get Fit and Provide Beauty and Healthful Bounty for Your Family

https://www.createspace.com/5459564

The gym is a great place to stay fit during the colder seasons, but once the temperature turns warmer you want to spend more time outside. Plus, you'll have the benefit of fresh wholesome produce to enjoy by growing vegetables in your backyard garden.

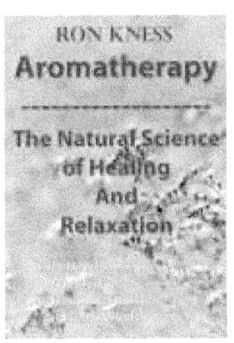

Aromatherapy - The Science of Healing and Relaxation: Learn How Essential Oils Elicit The Relaxation Response And Alter Mood

https://www.createspace.com/5714434

In my book Aromatherapy – The Science of Healing and Relaxation, we reveal the natural holistics methods you can use to heal the body from certain medical issues and to relive stress through relaxation. In particular we talk about:
• Aromatherapy - what it is and how it works

• Essential Oils – how the effects of certain aromas differs from others
• Recipes – how to make your own essential oil combinations

About the Author

I grew up in Central Minnesota, where my parents own and operated a fishing resort. Once out of high school I tried a couple of semesters of college, only to quit halfway through the Spring term; I decided at that time that college wasn't for me.

Then I decided to follow my father's previous occupation as an auto mechanic. I graduated from a two-year of vocational training course and worked as a mechanic. While in vocational training, I decided to join the National Guard where I eventually ended up working full-time for 32 years.

So how does all of this relate to writing? In one of my leadership schools, the instructor, who was an English teacher at a juvenile detention center, presented writing to me in a whole new way - a way that started to develop my interest in working with words.

Fast forward about 40 years and I now have over 50 books listed on Amazon for Kindle and CreateSpace.

Besides my own writing, I also ghostwrite ebooks, reports, articles, blogs and do Kindle conversions for my clients on a variety of topics.

Today my wife and I live in Gold Canyon, AZ, where you'll find me happily sitting in my office typing away on my laptop as I work on my next book or ghostwriting project . . . that is if we are not traveling on a cruise ship - our new-found mode of travel.

If you like my book, please leave a review of it.